Protein For Weight Loss

How protein can help you lose weight

By PROSENCE

publisher for any reparation, damages, or monetary loss due to the information herein, either directly or indirectly.

Respective authors own all copyrights not held by the publisher.

The information herein is offered for informational purposes solely, and is universal as so. The presentation of the information is without contract or any type of guarantee assurance.

The trademarks that are used are without any consent, and the publication of the trademark is without permission or backing by the trademark owner. All trademarks and brands within this book are for clarifying purposes only and are the owned by the owners themselves, not affiliated with this document.

ABOUT PROSENCE

Our Mission

We are dedicated to guiding, motivating and providing the tools necessary to transform people into the best version of themselves. Our goal is to empower men and women across the globe to realize that physical and mental fitness are not a short-term solution, but a lifetime choice, and to actualize what they have come to understand into a daily routine. We invite you to discover this process for yourself as you join us in the exploration of science-based knowledge that can lead to better health, greater fulfillment and astonishing vitality.

Who is Prosence?

Hi, I'm Antonio Mazzotta - certified Fitness Trainer and health enthusiast, and the founder of Prosence. While I don't think I'll ever turn down mom's homemade pasta and pizza, as an Italian living in Switzerland I've built a life dedicated to health and fitness. Now, I want to share the secrets to my success with you.

I got involved in this industry over 7 years ago, and quickly developed a passion for all things health and fitness. I knew right away that this is what I was born to do and haven't looked back. My days are spent developing new routines, training hard and meeting other fitness-minded and health-conscious individuals. I love working with my clients and coaching about weight training, dieting and healthy lifestyle choices. My number one priority is motivating people to achieve any fitness goal they seek. Whether you're looking to lose weight, get stronger, build cardio and endurance or just maintain overall health and vitality - I'm here to get you to your goals.

My team and I work hard to dispel the health and fitness myths and misinformation clogging the Internet today. We're driven by the desire to offer you a safe and manageable yet powerfully effective path to the best health of your life. Prosence is firmly committed to motivating, inspiring, and educating through the sharing of objective, fact-based health and fitness information that is rooted in science. We give you the tools you need to get in great shape and build a lifetime of good health.

Join us - let's work together to maximize your potential and achieve your optimal self while embracing life to the fullest!

Learn more on our website: www.prosencefitness.com, blog and keep up with the daily education and motivation by liking us on Twitter, Facebook & Instagram @prosencefitness.

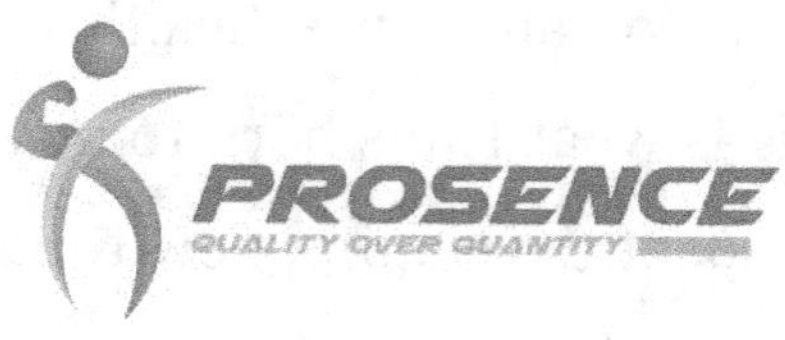

Table of Contents

Introduction

When looking to lose weight, people almost always turn to exercising without really committing to their diet. They do make slight changes to it, but oftentimes don't focus as much on maximizing their approach to dieting when contrasted with their approach to exercising. Assuming that applying common sense knowledge about dieting is all that you need to successfully lose weight/fat mass can be a big part of the reason you don't succeed in your weight loss journey.

The diet can be very complicated, with every small choice throughout the day impacting you physiologically and psychologically. Each macronutrient plays a vital role and can throttle your progress and chance at achieving your goal if you don't consume it appropriately. Luckily, common sense often dictates a few dietary rules in regards to carbohydrate and fat consumption that are easy to follow. But what about protein?

It's equally important and often not really considered or managed by those working on losing weight.

Keep on reading to become a pro at protein.

Chapter 1

What Does Protein Do?

Protein is a macronutrient. Macronutrients are nutrients that yield energy (contain calories) and are consumed in the diet. It is necessary for humans to consume large amounts of individual macronutrients for survival and adequate health.

Protein is composed of amino acids that can be broken down into individual components for use elsewhere in the body. The amino acid composition of protein can greatly differ, leading to variety in the quality and effects of proteins consumed.

Upon being consumed, protein can be broken down to serve several functions. Protein can facilitate the transport of other molecules within the body, act as enzymes for chemical reactions in the body, act as hormones, repair cells, and contribute to the growth of cells. It is recommended that protein be consumed in large amounts in the diet to allow for it to fill all of these roles. Even if someone is not an exerciser, it is necessary for their health to consume adequate amounts of high quality protein.

Protein is most commonly known for its role muscle protein synthesis (building muscle), and this function is arguably its most important for the exerciser. Consuming adequate amounts of protein allows for muscle to be both repaired and built post-exercise, which is very important. This is especially true for exercisers in a net caloric deficit who are attempting to lose weight. Being in a net caloric deficit means that an exerciser is consuming less calories than they are burning and is a prerequisite for significant fat loss. Given that immediately after exercising (especially resistance training) muscle protein breakdown is elevated, it is possible to lose muscle mass with training if under-consuming protein and attempting to lose weight (being in a net caloric deficit). However, the opposite can occur if consuming adequate amounts of protein. Some muscle mass can be built while attempting to lose fat mass if resistance training is included in an exerciser's training program. It is important to both spare and build muscle mass to facilitate fat loss because muscle tissue is more energetically expensive than fat tissue. This means that individuals with more muscle mass burn more calories, even at rest, than their counterparts with less muscle mass. This can facilitate fat loss by helping increase daily energy expenditure. Furthermore, the true goal of many exercisers attempting to lose weight isn't to actually lose weight. It's to improve their body composition. Doing so results in improved physical appearance, improved health, and improved relative strength.

To improve body composition an exerciser needs less fat mass and more fat free mass (such as muscle mass). Body composition is typically represented as a percentage value. The percentage indicates the percent of total body weight that is derived from fat mass. A bodyfat of 20% on a 100 lb person means they have 20 lbs of fat and 80 lbs of fat free mass. As an example, a man seeking to be lean enough to have visible abs might attempt to achieve the goal by losing 10 lbs, but they are actually trying to reach a point where their bodyfat is below 12%. This can be achieved by increasing muscle mass or thwarted by losing it. Exercisers who under-consume protein and are in a caloric deficit (causing muscle mass loss) are actually at risk of slowing their progress by increasing or maintaining their bodyfat percent, even with fat loss.

Though uncommon, protein can also be used for a process known as gluconeogenesis when the body is in a carbohydrate deprived state or when protein is overconsumed. Gluconeogenesis is the synthesis of glucose from another molecule or multiple other molecules. Glucose is typically derived from carbohydrates and is a very important energy substrate in the body. It is the primary source of fuel for a majority of exercise related tasks. Glucose is broken down to allow for energy production in both anaerobic (short duration, high intensity) and aerobic (long duration, low intensity) conditions. Glucose can even be used to fuel the brain, being one of the only large energy yielding macromolecules able to pass through the blood brain barrier. Its important functions can sustain physical activity and assist in the maintenance of physical activity over a long period of time. When glycogen (a stored form of glucose) runs low, physical activity becomes less sustainable. Consuming enough protein to help produce glucose in a pinch where carbohydrates and glycogen are running low can be beneficial to long duration exercise performance.

Given protein plays a role in gluconeogenesis, some rationalize that this would promote the feasibility of low carb or ketogenic diets. Though there is a time and place for both, it is typically not ideal to perform either extreme dietary measure. A vast majority of available research and basic logic do not support this fitness trend given the relationships between exercise intensity, exercise duration, blood glucose, insulin, and glycogen stores. Additionally, substrates necessary for aerobic respiration get removed from the krebs cycle to facilitate the production of ketone bodies. In doing this, aerobic respiration can be impeded decreasing exercise performance. Furthermore, the muscle sparing anti-catabolic effects of carbohydrates and insulin secretion are limited when under-consumed or not consumed at all. Though almost recommended, if considering whether a low carb or ketogenic diet is right for them, an exerciser should consult with a registered dietitian and sports nutritionist for a personalized evaluation and recommendation.

Protein has a variety of roles in the body, and many of them relate to exercise or exercise-related outcomes.

Chapter 2

Where Does Protein Come From?

The magnitude and type of effects that protein has on the body vary based on the exact protein consumed and different qualities/types of protein come from different sources. Not all proteins are created equal since amino acid composition of proteins can vary greatly. The quality of protein is mostly determined by the number of essential, conditionally essential, and nonessential amino acids that make up the macronutrient.

Essential amino acids are those that the body does not produce naturally on its own. They are necessary for survival and the regular healthy function of bodily systems given they can only be obtained through the diet. Conditionally essential amino acids are usually produced by the body and therefore do not need to be consumed in the diet for healthy function. But certain stressors and diseases are known to limit the number produced in the body, requiring them to be consumed in the diet instead. Nonessential amino acids are always produced by the body and don't need to be consumed in the diet for regular healthy function.

Generally, most individuals benefit from consuming complete proteins whether they exercise or not. Complete proteins are those that contain all 9 essential amino acids. Though given that all proteins consumed get broken down into their individual amino acids to be used in specific bodily processes, it is possible to consume two incomplete proteins that combined have all 9 essential amino acids and experience a similar effect to consuming one complete protein. It is easy to keep track of whether a protein is complete or incomplete because protein derived from specific sources almost always has the same composition.

Animal protein and dairy protein (e.g. milk, cheese, and yogurt) are complete protein sources. Fruit, vegetable, grain, and legume proteins are incomplete protein sources. Soy protein is a complete protein source but is unique in that its usefulness for exercisers is unknown. Some research supports its use and others claim its consumption is counterproductive. It is best to typically be safe and stay away from soy protein given the potential but unclear benefits aren't worth the potential and unclear drawbacks.

It is typically more convenient for most exercisers to consume animal and dairy proteins given they are often very protein dense, meaning they contain more protein per 100 calories than most other sources. Furthermore, muscle protein synthesis is most linked to the amino acid Leucine. This amino acid is typically found in highest concentrations in animal and dairy protein. Once a certain amount of leucine (in the form of a complete protein with other essential amino acids) has been consumed, muscle protein synthesis is maximized. Foods that are more leucine dense require less overall grams of protein to be consumed to yield an optimal effect. As an example, milk is more leucine dense than chicken, meaning it takes more chicken to maximize muscle protein synthesis than it would milk. This is an important consideration for the sake of feasibility in any diet. Having to consume more overall calories in a diet to maximize the effects of protein can be counterproductive and make it harder to lose weight. Additionally, it is more cost effective to get more bang for an exerciser's buck when purchasing food. The less they need to consume for their diet, the more money they end up being able to save. But, if unable or unwilling to consume animal and dairy proteins (e.g. because of availability, desire for variety, ethics, or religion), then it is completely reasonable to obtain protein through incomplete sources. But if this is done, they should be combined in a way that leads to the consumption of all essential amino acids within a meal. To do this, grains must simply be consumed with legumes during the same meal. Though it will likely be difficult to hit daily protein consumption goals with exclusively non-animal and non-dairy protein sources given they tend to be far less protein dense. Restrictive diets can also lead to boredom requiring creativity.

Protein can come from a variety of sources that influence its quality, but ultimately protein in one form or another can be found in nearly every food. There are trace amounts of protein in most foods consumed, even oreos.

Chapter 3

How Much Protein Do You Need?

Protein needs for individuals vary based on their level and type of physical activity as well as other factors in their diet and their health status. Though there can be alot of variety, the US FDA has made specific recommendations for the average healthy adult, though there is contention surrounding their recommendations.

The recommended daily allowance of protein intake is .8 grams per kg of bodyweight or .36 grams per lb of bodyweight. This recommendation is made for healthy adult males and females. Though the institute of medicine (IOM) proposes that between 10 to 35 percent of calories consumed in a day should come from protein in the average healthy adult male or female. Given that 1 gram of protein yields about 4 calories on average, the number of grams of protein consumed per day should be multiplied by 4 to determine the amount of calories consumed that come from protein. As an example, if an average healthy adult female consumes 2000 calories in her day and 100 grams of protein, 400 calories come from protein (100 x 4) and that equals 20% of her daily caloric intake (400 / 2000). This would put her within the range recommended by the institute of medicine.

The values recommended by the RDA (.8 grams per kg and .36 grams per lb) are controversial in that there is a lot of strong research supporting that this amount is not enough to allow for optimal adaptations to exercise stress and fully support a healthy musculoskeletal system. The RDA should be considered an absolute bare minimum rather than a target or a maximum intake. Protein recommendations do vary based on several factors, but the NSCA makes several recommendations based on training type and status. They recommend that exercisers in an aerobic endurance program (cardio based program) consume between 1 to 1.6 grams of protein per kg bodyweight (.45 to .72 grams per lb bodyweight) and that exercisers in a resistance training program (lifting based) consume between 1.4 to 1.7 grams of protein per kg bodyweight (.63 to .77 grams per lb of bodyweight). Though they also argue that most exercisers in a general fitness program can meet their goals by consuming between .8 to 1 grams of protein per kg bodyweight (.36 to .45 grams per lb of bodyweight). It is typically completely safe for a healthy individual to consume up to 2.1 grams of protein per kg bodyweight (.95 grams per lb of bodyweight), so even at the highest ranges of the recommendations made, an exerciser will not approach a risky amount of protein consumption. Individuals in muscle building and fat loss routines should typically consume an amount of protein on the higher end to promote muscle growth and muscle sparing. Consuming enough protein can also help facilitate bone growth and offset later life osteoporosis prematurely.

As mentioned earlier though, it is important that protein consumed be high quality and all amino acids be consumed in each meal. Otherwise the amount of protein consumed might have a lesser anabolic effect and be less helpful in muscle gain/sparing and subsequently fat loss/body composition improvement.

It is important to remember that all recommendations made by referenced bodies and organizations are intended solely for healthy adults and that those with clinically significant medical issues should consult with a registered dietitian and sports nutritionist.

When attempting to reach a protein goal or target in a diet, it is important to prioritize getting protein from non-supplement sources. The supplement industry isn't well regulated by the FDA and can thereby make misleading claims and subpar products. It is very common for supplements to be less effective at helping exercisers reach their goal than their whole food equivalent. Though there are some supplements with strong scientific support, their contents can still be consumed through the typical diet. As an example, whey protein has a high concentration of the amino acid leucine, which causes it to have a strong effect on muscle protein synthesis. But, milk also contains whey protein and has a similar effect. Typically actual food is more productive because consumption of it yields many benefits rather than a small host of them. For example consuming steak can provide a large amount of high quality protein, a medium amount of fat, a small amount of carbohydrates, creatine, the electrolyte sodium, and other vitamins and minerals. Consuming a whey isolate protein shake provides whey protein. Eating whole food provides a more comprehensive host of benefits instead of a small number of isolated benefits. Additionally, whole food tends to be cheaper long term given it provides many dietary nutrients that support or indirectly promote muscle building along with its protein. If supplements were bought to manage every need, it would be very pricey. Supplements are called supplements because they help exercisers meet dietary needs that they can't full satisfy through their diet, but that are being partially satisfied through their diet. Which means it is okay to consume whey protein if one is struggling to hit their protein target, but it should be more of a last resort than a first step.

Additionally given the lack of regulation in the supplement industry, cost-cutting companies, and sneaky advertising, alot of protein shakes available may have less potent anabolic effects than simply consuming a cup of milk. Some brands are more refined, but many are not given there are so many competing companies in the current market. Though if interested just for the taste or experience, it is rare that a whey protein shake would have a severe adverse effect. But, as mentioned earlier, soy protein is a bit sketchy given there is a large body of conflicting research. It is best to avoid it. Finally, if a protein shake of any type were consumed, it would typically be best to consume it immediately following the completion of a workout. Given it is a period where the body is most susceptible to muscle protein synthesis because of the hormonal responses to exercise, protein shakes (or really any high protein food) would be most effective if consumed then. It can also lead to muscle sparing because it is also the period where muscle breakdown is elevated. When consuming a large amount of protein post-workout, the subsequent insulin release, tissue repair, and positive net nitrogen balance can significantly help out an exerciser with their weight loss or body composition goals. It may be a useful strategy to save a good chunk of one's daily protein intake to be consumed immediately following a workout.

Chapter 4

Proteins Effect On Satiety

Adequate consumption of protein can also have a host of psychological benefits related to satiety. Satiety is the sensation of fullness one experiences when eating a meal. It is an important feeling as it is a naturally evolved mechanism for weight maintenance. If full, it is harder to consume more food and less likely. Many individuals eat until they feel full, but fullness isn't based exclusively on the amount of calories consumed, it is based on the type of food eaten.

Research supports that higher protein meals lead to greater satiety and less feelings of hunger. This is in part due to signaling that occurs from the gut to the brain when protein is digested. Given the psychological nature of eating, it is important for exercisers to have as many things in their favor as possible. Behavioral adherence to weight loss is extremely difficult for many, and a majority of those attempting to lose weight do not succeed because of this. It is oftentimes not due entirely to the actual behaviors engaged in, because if an exerciser is doing something relatively healthy they tend to progress in some form early on regardless of how slow. Though most do not bear with what they're doing long enough to see tangible results or do not engage in the most efficient methods of fat loss. If more psychologically motivated to engage in positive health behaviors, adherence would increase and more exerciser's goals would be met.

A strategy when eating can be to consume foods that are more protein rich earlier on. Doing this before getting to other foods in a meal that are sources of carbs or fat can help cause feelings of satiety before overeating occurs. Because there is a delay between the time food is eaten and satiety is signaled, it is possible for individuals eating fast to over-consume before recognizing they are no longer hungry. Another benefit to eating protein early and ensuring satiety signals come earlier on is that there's a tendency for protein rich foods to be rougher and take longer to eat than carbohydrate dense foods. It's easier to eat a ton of rice, pasta, or mashed potatoes really quickly. But it's hard to eat a chicken breast or turkey quickly. This can allow for even more of a buffer time between when food is consumed earlier on in a meal and satiety signals. It's especially important to allow for signals time to be sent when hungry. Being hungry makes it easier for one's eyes to be bigger than their stomach and lead to fast eating and high volume eating. Both are counterproductive for weight loss. Ironically, those that are trying to lose weight often go through periods of little food consumption in an attempt to limit their caloric intake. This eventually makes them very hungry at the start of their meals and increases the likelihood of poor eating behaviors. This is why it's even more important to signal satiety early on. Though, aside from early meal protein consumption, consuming water at the start of a meal can help lead to further satiety later in the meal. The more water that gets consumed, the more full someone generally feels during a meal.

Chapter 5

List Of Protein Rich Foods

There are dozens of protein rich foods out there to be consumed and it would be impractical to list them all, but some of the best are listed below.

Complete Proteins:
1. Eggs
2. Greek Yogurt
3. Milk
4. Cottage Cheese
5. Chicken Breasts
6. Tuna
7. Jerky
8. Swiss Cheese
9. Beef
10. Turkey Breasts
11. Shrimp
12. Pork
13. Steak

14. Whey Protein Shakes

Incomplete Proteins:
1. Quinoa
2. Peanuts
3. Peanut Butter
4. Almonds
5. Lentils
6. Broccoli
7. Kidney Beans

Chapter 6

Frequently Asked Questions

I'm a vegan, am I at a significant disadvantage because of this?

The unfortunate answer is that those with vegan dietary preferences kind of are at a bit of a disadvantage. Given the psychological nature of dietary health behavior, having a near infinite variety of options allows for the development of many strategies to help exercisers lose weight. The less tools (food types) there are to work with, the less flexibility there is to problem solve and find ways to increase adherence to a weight loss diet. Additionally, creatine is found in high concentrations in some meats and can promote muscle building and workout intensity which both facilitate fat loss. Furthermore most leucine rich high protein foods come from animal products which can mean vegan exercisers might have to consume more grams of protein than their animal product consuming counterparts. Though there are additional difficulties vegans may have to overcome, it is still very plausible for them to combine incomplete proteins at each meal and facilitate weight loss and muscle building/sparing. They just have to be more careful. Their fitness goals can still be achieved while adhering to their dietary preferences and belief system.

Aside from the mention of protein ingestion post-workout, are there any other tips or tricks related to protein consumption timing I should be aware of?

In general, the timing of protein consumption won't affect all too much for the typical exerciser from a physiological standpoint. It is still beneficial to consume more protein around the workout period for the effects earlier described. Though, from a satiety and psychological standpoint, it can be beneficial to consume moderate amounts of protein at consistent intervals throughout the day. This can prevent an exerciser from feeling overly hungry at the start of their meals and thereby preemptively curb tendencies to overeat. Though it should be noted that it isn't necessary to consume protein at regular intervals. If an individual finds they are best able to adhere to their diet and eat reasonable amounts of food by consuming protein at less frequent timestamps then they should continue to do what works best for them. Also, from a practical standpoint, there is no need to worry about over-consuming protein in a single meal if daily protein intake is still within recommended ranges. Most will not reach a dangerous level of protein consumption within a single meal.

Does it matter if I really like one source of complete protein and consume that for most of my protein needs?

In terms of muscle protein synthesis and the other positive weight loss facilitating effects of protein consumption, it is typically fine to consume a majority of one's daily protein from a single source. This is provided they also consume a variety of other foods to allow for appropriate vitamin and mineral consumption. Having less diverse diets can lead to difficulties consuming certain nutrients and lead to deficiencies so it is important to supplement the consumption of one main protein source with many other types of foods for the rest of that individual's macronutrient goals. Generally though, if possible, it is safer to consume multiple types of complete protein throughout the typical date. Even if both have all the essential amino acids, one probably has less of certain amino acids. The other source of protein can make up for it.

Will over consuming protein lead to kidney damage?

It is possible for renal function to be impaired by over-consuming protein. But it is very difficult to do so and one would have to consume over 3 times (300%) the recommended daily allowance of protein to be at risk of this occurring. So it is not a practical consideration for a healthy adult as long as they stay within the scope of what organizations like the NSCA, US FDA, and IOM recommend.

Conclusion

I hope that this protein guide will in some way serve to provide all of you out there with the foundation for future success. It can be hard to accomplish your goals if your diet isn't in check. Every little thing you do will count and influence you physiologically, psychologically, or both.

Seeing as we've reached the end of our journey, it's important that you use the information you've learned here to shape your diet and your future lean body. It's really easy to go out there and buy the right protein rich foods for your needs. You have a ton of options at your fingertips and can eat with purpose now.

Thank you for purchasing this book, I hope you enjoyed it.

Finally, if you enjoyed this book then I'd like to ask you for a favor. Will you be kind enough to leave a review for this book on Amazon? It would be greatly appreciated!

Don't forget to follow us on Twitter, Facebook & Instagram and visit our website www.prosencefitness.com to get empowered, educated and inspired to become the best version of yourself in life! You deserve it.

References

1. Haff, G., & Triplett, N. T. (2016). Essentials of strength training and conditioning. Champaign, IL: Human Kinetics.

2. Westerterp-Plantenga, M. S., Nieuwenhuizen, A., Tome, D., Soenen, S., & Westerterp, K. R. (2009). Dietary protein, weight loss, and weight maintenance. *Annual review of nutrition, 29*, 21-41.

3. Phillips, S. M. (2006). Dietary protein for athletes: from requirements to metabolic advantage. *Applied physiology, nutrition, and metabolism, 31*(6), 647-654.

4. Westerterp-Plantenga, M. S., Lemmens, S. G., & Westerterp, K. R. (2012). Dietary protein—its role in satiety, energetics, weight loss and health. *British journal of nutrition, 108*(S2), S105-S112.

5. Kreider, R. B., & Campbell, B. (2009). Protein for exercise and recovery. *The Physician and sportsmedicine, 37*(2), 13-21.

6. Gilbert, J. A., Bendsen, N. T., Tremblay, A., & Astrup, A. (2011). Effect of proteins from different sources on body composition. *Nutrition, Metabolism and Cardiovascular Diseases, 21*, B16-B31.